Overweight dispose

"Shedding Pounds: Effective Strategies for Overweight Disposal"

By

2023 by Ago Winnie

program, always consult your
doctor or another licensed
healthcare professional.

Cover design by Ago Winnie

Table of contents

Introduction

Overweight disposal is a critical issue that affects individuals, communities, and societies at large. It refers to the process of effectively managing and addressing the problem of overweight or obesity. With the global prevalence of overweight and obesity on the rise, it is essential to focus on

implementing strategies that promote healthy lifestyles and sustainable weight loss.

Firstly, overweight disposal is crucial for individual well-being. Excessive weight can lead to a range of health problems, including heart disease, diabetes, and joint issues. By actively working towards weight loss and maintenance, individuals can significantly reduce the risk of developing such conditions and improve their overall quality of life. This includes adopting a balanced and nutritious diet, engaging in regular physical activity, and seeking professional guidance and support.

Moreover, overweight disposal positively impacts communities. When individuals strive to achieve and maintain a healthy weight, they contribute to the creation of healthier and more vibrant communities. Reduced overweight and obesity rates can lead to lower healthcare costs, increased productivity, and improved social cohesion. Additionally, communities that prioritize healthy living and weight management can offer more opportunities for physical activity, such as parks, recreational facilities, and active transportation options.

On a larger scale, society benefits from effective overweight disposal strategies. By investing in prevention programs and education, societies can combat the economic burden of obesity-related healthcare costs. Moreover, promoting healthy lifestyles and weight management fosters a culture of wellness, empowering individuals to make informed choices about their health and well-being. This, in turn, helps create a society that values and prioritizes preventive healthcare, leading to a healthier and more resilient population.

In conclusion, overweight disposal is an essential aspect of promoting individual, community, and societal well-being. By adopting healthy lifestyles, individuals can reduce their risk of chronic diseases, enhance their quality of life, and contribute to healthier communities. Furthermore, societies that prioritize overweight disposal strategies can reap the economic and social benefits associated with a healthier population. Through collective efforts, education, and support, we can effectively address the challenge of overweight and obesity, paving the way for a healthier future.

CHAPTER 1:

what is overweight and why is it a problem .

Overweight refers to a condition in which a person carries excess body weight, primarily due to an accumulation of fat. It is typically determined by calculating the body mass index (BMI), which considers a person's weight in relation to their height. An individual with a BMI of 25 to 29.9 is classified as overweight, while a BMI of 30 or above is classified as obese.

Overweight is a significant problem with wide-ranging consequences for individuals and society as a whole. Firstly, it poses serious health risks. Excess weight increases the likelihood of developing chronic conditions such as heart disease, type 2 diabetes, high blood pressure, certain cancers, and respiratory problems. Overweight individuals are also prone to musculoskeletal disorders and experience a reduced quality of life due to limited mobility and physical discomfort.

Furthermore, being overweight can have detrimental effects on mental health. It often leads to low self-esteem, body image issues, and depression. Overweight individuals may face societal stigmatization, discrimination, and social exclusion, which further exacerbate their mental well-being.

The economic impact of overweight is substantial. Healthcare costs rise due to the increased prevalence of chronic diseases associated with excess weight. This places a burden on healthcare systems and can strain resources. Additionally, overweight individuals may experience decreased work productivity and face discrimination in the job market, leading to financial implications for both individuals and society.

Childhood overweight is particularly concerning. It sets the stage for a lifelong struggle with weight management and can have lasting physical and psychological effects. Overweight children are at a higher risk of becoming overweight adults, perpetuating the cycle of health problems and societal costs.

Addressing overweight requires a multifaceted approach. Promoting healthy eating habits, regular physical activity, and lifestyle changes are crucial. Public health campaigns, education, and access to nutritious foods play vital roles in preventing and managing overweight. Moreover, support from healthcare professionals, communities, and policy-makers is necessary to create environments that encourage healthy choices and combat the systemic factors contributing to overweight.

In conclusion, overweight is a pervasive and complex problem with significant health, social, and economic consequences. By recognizing its impact and implementing comprehensive strategies, we can work towards healthier societies, improved well-being, and a reduced burden on individuals and healthcare systems.

CHAPTER 2:

The Dangers of Overweight

The dangers of overweight or obesity cannot be overstated in today's society. As the prevalence of this condition continues to rise at an alarming rate, it is crucial to understand the significant risks and potential consequences associated with carrying excess weight. From physical to psychological complications, the dangers of overweight affect individuals on multiple levels, impacting both their quality and length of life.

One of the most immediate dangers of overweight is its impact on physical health. Carrying excess weight puts immense strain on the body's systems, leading to an increased risk of chronic diseases such as heart disease, type 2 diabetes, hypertension, and certain types of cancer. These conditions can have severe implications for one's well-being, often resulting in reduced mobility, decreased life expectancy, and a diminished overall quality of life.

Furthermore, overweight individuals are more likely to experience musculoskeletal problems, including joint pain, osteoarthritis, and back issues. The additional weight places excessive pressure on bones and joints, leading to long-term damage and reduced mobility. Additionally, overweight individuals often suffer from respiratory difficulties, sleep apnea, and decreased lung function, exacerbating the risks to their overall health.

Beyond the physical dangers, overweight also takes a toll on mental and emotional well-being. Individuals struggling with weight issues often face societal stigmatization, leading to body image concerns, low self-esteem, and increased risk of depression and anxiety. Social isolation and discrimination can further exacerbate these psychological effects, creating a vicious cycle that negatively impacts overall mental health.

The dangers of overweight
extend beyond individual
well-being, also affecting
society as a whole. The
economic burden of obesity is
substantial, with increased
healthcare costs and lost
productivity due to related
health issues. Additionally, the
strain on healthcare systems
can limit resources and access
for other individuals in need.

In conclusion, the dangers of
overweight are multifaceted,
impacting physical, mental,
and societal well-being. It is
imperative to prioritize

preventive measures such as healthy eating habits, regular physical activity, and access to quality healthcare. By addressing the dangers of overweight, we can improve the overall health and well-being of individuals and work towards building a healthier society.

CHAPTER 3:

Benefits and risks of weight loss surgery

Weight loss surgery, also known as bariatric surgery, has become an increasingly popular option for individuals struggling with obesity. While it offers numerous benefits, it is important to consider the

potential risks as well. Here are the key advantages and risks associated with weight loss surgery.

Benefits:
1. Significant and sustained weight loss: Weight loss surgery can help individuals achieve substantial and long-lasting weight loss, leading to improved overall health and a reduced risk of obesity-related conditions such as joint issues, diabetes, and cardiovascular disease.

2. Resolution of obesity-related health conditions: Many individuals who undergo weight loss surgery experience significant improvements or complete resolution of conditions like type 2 diabetes, sleep apnea, high blood pressure, and high cholesterol.

3. Enhanced quality of life: Losing excess weight can improve physical mobility, increase energy levels, and boost self-esteem and body image. It can also lead to a

greater sense of well-being and improved social interactions.

4. Increased lifespan: By reducing the risk of obesity-related health problems, weight loss surgery has the potential to extend an individual's lifespan and improve their overall health trajectory.

Risks:
1. Surgical complications: Like any major surgery, weight loss surgery carries risks such as infection, bleeding, blood clots, and adverse reactions to

anesthesia. These risks can vary depending on the specific procedure performed.

2. Nutritional deficiencies: Following weight loss surgery, individuals may be at risk of developing nutritional deficiencies due to reduced food intake and malabsorption. Regular monitoring and appropriate dietary supplements can help mitigate this risk.

3. Gallstones: Rapid weight loss after surgery can increase the likelihood of developing

gallstones, which may require additional treatment such as medication or surgical removal.

4. Psychological and emotional challenges: Weight loss surgery is not a cure-all solution and individuals may face psychological and emotional challenges as they adjust to their new lifestyle. These may include body image issues, relationship changes, and the need for ongoing support and counseling.

In conclusion, weight loss surgery offers significant benefits for individuals struggling with obesity, including substantial weight loss, resolution of obesity-related health conditions, and an improved quality of life. However, it is essential to acknowledge and address the potential risks associated with the surgical procedure, including surgical complications, nutritional deficiencies, gallstones, and psychological challenges. It is crucial for individuals considering weight loss

surgery to have a thorough
understanding of both the
benefits and risks, and to
consult with a healthcare
professional to make an
informed decision.

CHAPTER 4:

Choosing a weight loss medication

Choosing a weight loss medication can be a significant decision in one's journey towards a healthier lifestyle. With the abundance of options available in the market, it's essential to make an informed choice that aligns with your

specific needs and goals. Consider the following factors when selecting a weight loss medication to ensure you make the right decision.

Firstly, consult a healthcare professional. Seeking guidance from a medical expert is crucial as they can evaluate your overall health, assess potential risks, and recommend the most suitable medication for your individual circumstances. They will consider factors such as your body mass index (BMI), medical history, and any existing conditions to determine the appropriate course of action.

Additionally, carefully review the medication's safety profile and effectiveness. Look for medications that have undergone rigorous clinical trials and have been approved by reputable regulatory authorities. Examine the potential side effects, contraindications, and precautions associated with the medication to ensure its compatibility with your health status.

Consider the mode of action of the medication. Some weight loss medications work by suppressing appetite, while others focus on inhibiting fat absorption or increasing metabolism. Choose a medication that addresses your specific weight loss needs and aligns with your preferred approach to managing your weight.

Furthermore, take into account the lifestyle changes required alongside the medication. Weight loss medications should complement a balanced diet and regular physical activity. Ensure that you are willing and able to make the necessary lifestyle adjustments to support the medication's effectiveness.

Cost is another crucial factor. Evaluate the affordability of the medication, including any potential insurance coverage or assistance programs. Keep in mind that weight loss medications may need to be taken for an extended period, so it's essential to choose an

option that fits within your
budget.

In conclusion, selecting a
weight loss medication is a
decision that should be made
in consultation with a
healthcare professional.
Consider factors such as
safety, effectiveness, mode of
action, lifestyle changes, and
cost to make an informed
choice. Remember that weight
loss medications should be
part of a comprehensive
approach that includes a
healthy diet, regular exercise,
and ongoing medical

supervision. By carefully evaluating these factors, you can choose a weight loss medication that supports your journey towards a healthier weight and improved well-being.

Chapter 5:

Approaches to Overweight Disposal

Overweight and obesity have become a significant health concern in many parts of the world. With sedentary lifestyles and unhealthy dietary habits on the rise, finding effective approaches to overweight disposal is crucial for individuals looking to improve their well-being. Here are some key strategies that can help in the battle against excess weight.

1. Balanced Diet: Adopting a balanced and nutritious diet is fundamental in achieving weight loss goals. Focus on consuming whole foods, such as fruits, vegetables, lean proteins, and whole grains. Avoid processed foods high in sugar, unhealthy fats, and empty calories. Portion control is also important, as it helps regulate calorie intake.

2. Regular Physical Activity: Engaging in regular exercise is essential for weight management. Incorporate a combination of aerobic

exercises, such as jogging, swimming, or cycling, with strength training to build muscle and boost metabolism. Aim for at least 150 minutes of moderate-intensity activity per week, along with strength training exercises twice a week.

3. Behavior Modification: Adopting healthy behaviors and making sustainable lifestyle changes is crucial for long-term weight management. Identify triggers for overeating or unhealthy habits and develop strategies

to overcome them. Setting realistic goals and tracking progress can help stay motivated and focused on the weight loss journey.

4. Mindful Eating: Practicing mindful eating involves paying attention to physical hunger and fullness cues, as well as being aware of the emotions and environmental factors influencing eating behaviors. Slow down while eating, savor each bite, and listen to your body's signals to prevent overeating.

5. Support Systems: Seeking support from friends, family, or professionals can make a significant difference in weight loss efforts. Joining a weight loss group, seeking guidance from a registered dietitian, or working with a personal trainer can provide the necessary accountability, motivation, and knowledge to achieve success.

6. Stress Management: Chronic stress can contribute to weight gain. Finding healthy ways to manage stress, such as through exercise, meditation,

or engaging in hobbies, can help prevent emotional eating and support overall well-being.

Remember, every individual is unique, and it may take time to find the approach that works best for you. Consult with healthcare professionals or registered dietitians for personalized guidance based on your specific needs and health conditions.

By combining these approaches to overweight disposal, individuals can embark on a journey toward a healthier weight and improved overall health and well-being. Persistence, patience, and consistency are key to achieving and maintaining a healthy weight in the long term.

CHAPTER 6:

Building an exercise routine

Building an exercise routine can be an effective way to

improve your physical and mental health. However, starting a new fitness routine can be overwhelming, especially if you are new to exercise. Here are some steps you can take to build a successful exercise routine.

1. Set a Goal: The first step in building an exercise routine is to determine your goal. Do you want to lose weight, build muscle, improve your flexibility, or simply improve your overall fitness? Once you have a goal in mind, you can

create a plan that will help you achieve it.

2. Choose the Right Activities: Once you have set a goal, choose the activities that will help you achieve it. Cardiovascular exercise, such as running, cycling, or swimming, can help you burn calories and improve your heart health. Strength training, such as weightlifting or bodyweight exercises, can help you build muscle and improve your overall strength. Yoga or Pilates can help you

improve your flexibility and reduce stress.

3. Start Slowly: It's important to start slowly and gradually increase the intensity and duration of your workouts. If you are new to exercise, start with just a few minutes of activity each day and gradually increase the time and intensity.

4. Create a Schedule: Schedule your workouts at a time that is convenient for you. This will assist you in incorporating

exercise into your daily
routine.

**5. Track Your Progress: Keep
track of your progress by
recording your workouts,
tracking your weight or
measurements, or using a
fitness app or wearable device.
This will help you stay
motivated and see the progress
you are making.**

**6. Mix It Up: To avoid
boredom and plateauing, mix
up your workouts. Try
different activities, change the**

intensity, or add new exercises to your routine.

7. Get Support: Finally, get support from friends, family, or a personal trainer. Having someone to hold you accountable and offer encouragement can help you stay on track and reach your goals.

In conclusion, building an exercise routine takes time and effort, but it is worth it for the benefits it can bring to your physical and mental health. By setting a goal, choosing the right activities, starting slowly, creating a schedule, tracking your progress, mixing it up, and getting support, you can create a successful exercise routine that you can stick to for the long-term.

CHAPTER 7:

Strategies for maintaining weight loss

Maintaining weight loss can be a challenging endeavor, but with the right strategies, it is possible to sustain your progress and enjoy a healthier, happier lifestyle. Here are some key strategies to help you maintain weight loss successfully.

1. Adopt a Balanced and Sustainable Diet: Focus on incorporating whole, nutrient-dense foods into your diet, such as fruits, vegetables, lean proteins, whole grains, and healthy fats. Avoid extreme diets or strict restrictions, as they are often difficult to sustain long-term. Strive for moderation and portion control.

2. Regular Exercise: Physical activity is crucial for

maintaining weight loss. Exercise your heart, your muscles, and your flexibility at the same time. In order to make fitness a habit you can maintain, find something you like to do. In addition to muscle-strengthening exercises at least twice per week, aim for at least 150 minutes of moderate-intensity aerobic activity or 75 minutes of vigorous-intensity cardiovascular exercise per week.

3. Monitor Your Progress: Keep track of your weight,

food intake, and exercise routine. Regularly monitoring your progress can help you stay accountable and identify any potential setbacks before they become major obstacles.

4. Set Realistic Goals: Rather than focusing on a specific number on the scale, set goals related to overall health and well-being. Aim for weekly weight loss of 1-2 pounds and prioritize long-term lifestyle changes above temporary ones.

5. Build a Support System:
Surround yourself with a
supportive network of friends,
family, or a support group who
understand and encourage
your weight loss journey.
Having a support system can
provide motivation,
accountability, and guidance
during challenging times.

6. Practice Mindful Eating:
Pay attention to your hunger
and fullness cues, eat slowly,
and savor each bite. Avoid
distractions while eating, such
as watching TV or using
electronic devices. This helps

you develop a better
relationship with food and
prevents overeating.

7. Manage Stress: Stress can
lead to emotional eating and
hinder weight loss
maintenance efforts. Find
healthy ways to manage stress,
such as engaging in relaxation
techniques, practicing
mindfulness, getting enough
sleep, and engaging in
activities you enjoy.

8. Stay Hydrated: Drinking an
adequate amount of water can
help control cravings, support

digestion, and keep you feeling full. Aim to drink at least 8 cups of water per day.

9. Maintain a Consistent Routine: Stick to regular mealtimes and consistent sleep patterns. Having a structured routine helps regulate your body's hunger and fullness signals.

10. Celebrate Non-Scale Victories: Acknowledge and celebrate the non-scale victories along your journey, such as improved energy levels, increased strength, and better overall health.

Remember, maintaining weight loss is a lifelong commitment. Embrace a positive mindset, be patient with yourself, and focus on sustainable habits that support your long-term well-being. With these strategies in place, you can maintain your weight loss and enjoy a healthier and more fulfilling life.

Conclusion:

In conclusion, the issue of overweight disposal is one that demands urgent attention and comprehensive action. The consequences of this global epidemic are far-reaching, affecting individuals, communities, and societies as a whole. However, through education, awareness, and a commitment to promoting healthier lifestyles, we can

overcome the challenges posed
by overweight disposal and
create a healthier future.

First and foremost, it is crucial
to recognize that overweight
disposal is not simply a matter
of personal responsibility, but
a multifaceted problem that
requires a collective effort.
Governments, healthcare
professionals, educators, and
individuals all have a role to
play in addressing this issue.
By implementing policies that
promote access to nutritious
foods, encouraging physical
activity, and regulating the

marketing of unhealthy
products, governments can
create an environment that
supports healthy choices.
Additionally, healthcare
professionals can provide
guidance and support to
individuals struggling with
their weight, while educators
can integrate comprehensive
health and nutrition education
into school curricula.

Public awareness campaigns
also play a pivotal role in
combating overweight
disposal. By disseminating
accurate information about

the risks associated with obesity and the benefits of maintaining a healthy weight, we can empower individuals to make informed decisions about their health. Furthermore, these campaigns can help reduce the stigma and discrimination faced by overweight individuals, fostering a more inclusive and supportive society.

Addressing overweight disposal requires a long-term commitment to sustainable lifestyle changes. It is not about quick fixes or fad diets, but rather about fostering a culture of health and well-being. This includes promoting regular physical activity, cultivating healthy eating habits, and encouraging self-care practices that prioritize mental and emotional well-being.

In conclusion, the issue of overweight disposal is a complex challenge that demands a comprehensive and collaborative approach. By working together, we can create a society that values and supports healthy lifestyles, ensuring a brighter and healthier future for generations to come. It is only through collective action and sustained efforts that we can overcome the burden of overweight disposal and pave the way for a healthier and happier world.